Balance With Colour
Journal

Lorraine and Dr Bob Roberts PhD

Ordering Information:

Prime Seven Media
518 Landmann St.
Tomah City, WI 54660

Printed in the United States of America

Dedication

We want to dedicate this book to those people who are prepared to look at all possible ways to make a positive difference in the way they care for themselves, and who can be empathetic to everything on our planet Earth, because we all depend on each other in one way or another.

What you freely give

You lift my spirits, calm my nerves, and you ground me. At the same time, you also help bring me back to reality. No matter where you are moved to, you thrive, and you seem happy. You bring such joy into my life, and you reward me constantly for taking care of you. I love to visit you often, and you greet me with lovely smells and beautiful coloured flowers. A garden to care for surrounded by flowers, trees, herbs, and edible plants, to nurture just once in a while makes me feel so lucky. It is a privilege for me to share you with others so we can all benefit from your natural energy and beauty. To protect you from being invaded is a small price to pay because everyone needs what you can freely give. I will take care of you when I see you are surrounded by others wanting your space. We all appreciate the benefit that Nature has given us, knowing that later today, tomorrow or any day soon, you will fade away and may even die. But I will wait most patiently, knowing you may suddenly surprise me, and I see you are ready to grow back once again. I will stay as long as I can to greet you and take care of you . And if not me, there will be someone else, until you are there no more because they have moved you to make space for something else, a home or a road? Who knows!

Introduction

Journaling, meditation, mindfulness, and being grateful and empathetic have become increasingly more important for us to get our minds clear and to be aware of where we put our focus or how we use our energy: meaning, to get our thinking back into balance, and be positive, so that we do not become overwhelmed but are able to cope with our daily stresses.

From the beginnings of time, Nature has provided us (through our pure instincts) with positive messages on how to survive and prosper. We still have that instinct in our DNA but have sent it to the background. Meaning we have lost touch with our true nature and are now struggling to understand it and to get back to it. Being aware of what our body is telling us (being mindful); going with the natural order of day and night); relaxing in the sunshine; do meditation; and taking time to reflect (story-telling and journaling) that are all natural to us. One way for us to do this is to record our daily activities. We need time to focus inward and to completely relax and clear our minds. Routine, discipline and respect for self and others are also very important behavioural characteristics for our survival. But we need a tool to bring balance into our lives, and so the interpretation of the use of colour in Nature, based on how we perceive the positive messages colour in natural settings, that Nature has been sending us since the beginning of time, is so important. By focusing on the uplifting and positive messages that Nature provides and by using colour in Nature to remind us of those messages, we are able to be more in control of our emotions, thoughts, and actions. What we then notice is the flow-on effect that radiates to each other, so that if we are calm, for instance, we make people around us calm as well.

The Balance With Colour: To avoid sliding into depression book came to us from the desire to share this tool with anyone who has a need and wants to become more positive in their life, using colour in Nature that inspires positive messages to achieve balance in life.

For anyone who wants to share the Balance With Colour concept and technique, for the benefit of individuals or families, young or old, who would like to improve their confidence and self-worth, have empathy and to be more understanding towards others, refer to the Balance With Colour: Guide. Also included in the guidebook there are samples of the sets of bookmarks of various designs, and a simple meditation guide. Additionally, there is a set of cards, titled, Balance With Colour - Condensed Information and Cards; a set of Positive Focus Wristbands, which has one band of each colour that can be worn each day to remind the wearer of their commitment to a particular positive thought and action for that day. We have created two support novels: A Journey of Discovery, a story about how a family, working together, discovered Balance With Colour, and achieved balance in their family life, and Colour in Nature: And the positive messages and words that come to mind, a story about how a granddad shares the Balance With Colour concept and technique with his granddaughter and her group of friends. There are also complimentary support videos and a meditation video on YouTube, under the name Lorraine Roberts, Maju Publications.

Think carefully about how you feel when experiencing a colourful natural scene, just as early man would have seen and felt it. Those perceptions have enabled us to gain confidence and to focus on positive thoughts, words, and actions, and thus we have been able to solve or control any problems calmly and constructively that were overwhelming us and making us feel extremely stressed, anxious, fearful, and dysfunctional.

Our hope is that, as it has been for us, using the Balance With Colour: Journal, will help others to feel calm, in control, and to be more positive as they face their daily challenges. We wish the users the success that we are experiencing.

Lorraine and Bob
Rosemount
2022

Sadly, in this life we often take too much for granted, our health, family and friends, our culture, and our language.

Taken for granted

Our most treasured inheritance.
It is not gold we are talking about.
It is not money, a home or a fancy car.
Could it be something more precious **?**
Something we take for granted perhaps **?**
Something that could so easily be lost
And then quite difficult to get back **?**
You have to experience it to know.
But just imagine losing your land,
Or worst still your native language **?**
When language is your true identity,
To communicate, and be understood;
To sing songs you know rhyme nicely,
With words that easly roll off your tounge,
In a language that has been passed on
And you know where you belong.
Wouldn't you protect your language
And not ever take it for granted **?**

This poem is from Lorraine's book of poems, wise saying and short stories, When you think of it.... © 2018

Our languge is our history and we learn from history what is important and what we need to change. And so it is with Nature. You only have to look around and notice all that we take for granted. It is only when it is no longer there that we realise the importance of all that Nature has provided for us. But it is a two-way thing and can bounce back making it a win-win for all; and not only with Nature but with our relationships with each other as well. So it starts with self-improvement and we win in so many ways.

Why Colour?

Colour all around in Nature is a necessary part of life because that is how we distinguish what we see and from which we can get important messages. Since the beginning of time, we humans have had to rely on colour to inform us and to help us to survive.

We have gradually been able to duplicate the colours we see in Nature and use them to our advantage, as in knowing what benefits certain coloured foods provide for our wellbeing, and what to use as medicine, or even to persuade us to buy what is being offered to us. We choose certain colours because they make us feel good and maybe give us confidence, or as in a uniform, which can make us feel a sense of belonging or acceptance. We have favourite colours for some reason and even colours we dislike, only because we have had a bad experience associated with that colour or someone had told us that that colour will bring bad luck or represents evil. But the truth is, colour in Nature is there and it is there for a very good reason and all living beings benefit from colour in one way or another. What might be a warning of danger for one could actually be indicating another form of benefit to others. The important thing is to appreciate and study colour in Nature and to use those insights the way Nature meant them to be used. We live in a shared world relying on each other and so we need to protect and care for what Nature has provided for all to survive. We need to keep rejuvenating and replacing what we take from Nature because it is not only for our survival. Everything in moderation and in balance.

In Balance With Colour, we use colour to remind us to focus on the positive messages we get from colour in Nature to help us with our mental wellbeing and to manage our day-to-day stresses or to keep from becoming overwhelmed by problems that can make us overly anxious. Balance With Colour is not about colour therapy, it is simply about using colour in Nature (any colour) in a positive way to influence our thinking to enable us to cope with day-to-day stresses. In this way, a particular colour is not used to define the effects of that colour on any medical or psychological condition but rather to simply enable us to think of the positives instead of the negatives. It does not clash with but rather complements any religious or wellbeing programme anyone is already using. It is in no way going to cure or help us get over traumas or grief because they are caused by outside influences that we cannot control. If a person has already become clinically depressed, they may need professional help but can still use the Balance With Colour tool in addition to any other help they are receiving. What it does is enable us to control our emotional reactions. Balance With Colour is to prevent us sliding into depression.

The reason for choosing seven colours, green, blue, pink, yellow, red, white, and black, for the Balance With Colour technique is that that number fits in with using one particular colour for each day of the week to get us into the habit of using a colour to focus on a particular word for that day, for a whole week. However, other colours, such as grey, brown, purple, etc., can also be used if we regard them as a mix of two or more colours: grey being a mix of black and white, so we could choose either black or white to focus on the positive messages we get from seeing that colour in Nature; brown, being a mix of red and yellow, and so we could focus either on red or on yellow; purple, being a mix of red and blue, so focus either on red or on blue; lime green being yellow or green; orange being red or yellow; and so on. This is useful when choosing to use the orange colour in chakra healing to provide the energy associated with the healing needed using that colour so that the colour red or yellow in Nature can also be a reminder of the word or words we have chosen for that chakra healing. Another way it can help when using the chakra healing is if you have already chosen a particular colour because it has been set for that day, then choose that colour also to heal that particular part of your body.

Colour all around us and is a gift from Nature since the beginning of time. Colour can lift our spirits and feed our soul.

Imagine how the first humans might have seen colour for the first time. Colour as it still is today, that Nature had provided for them that must have excited them. How they reacted when the sun came up, and they saw a beautiful, clear blue sky; and how would the first humans have felt when they walked through a forest, which for us now might be like walking around a botanical garden? They would have walked the hot desert land and gone through different kinds of forests and noticed all the many colours: the green shoots in spring that mean new growth, life, and food. They would have worked out what it meant to see the sky red in the late afternoon; or to see the woods on fire when lightning stuck and noticed that the red flames were the same colour as that of their blood and whatever else they noticed was red. They would have seen the variety of coloured birds that would have delighted them, as would the colours that come together often after a storm in the form of a rainbow. They would have found uses for what was on offer in this beautiful colourful world and would not have had any negative association with colour. When colours changed with the seasons, they would have known to prepare themselves for what was to come and what there was to be enjoyed. They may have moved around and settled in different places to make themselves more comfortable, while tasting different coloured foods and enjoying the changed scenery. They would have noticed and tried to follow a rainbow, possibly looking for what could be at the end of a rainbow! Naturally, they would have had to have invented names for all the different colours, words to show their delight and to express their feelings and give meanings. Wise words and wisdom to pass on.

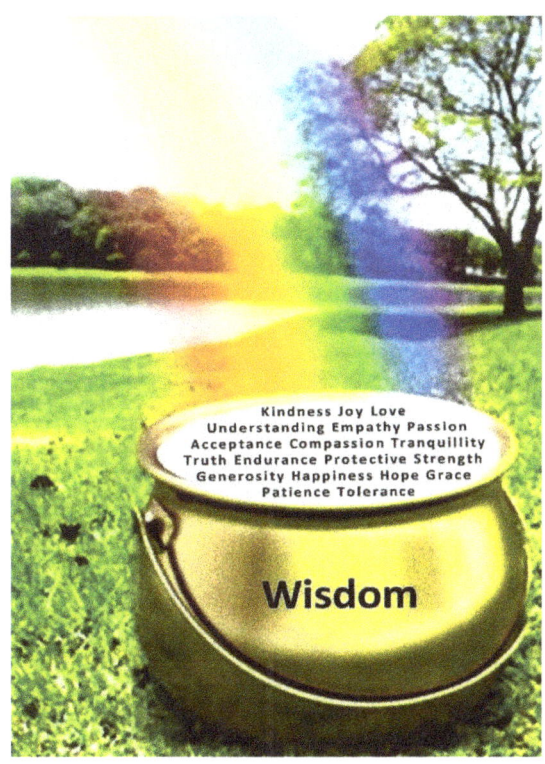

Wise words and messages we can still use today, a gift from Nature to lift our spirits.

Colour in Nature

Nature has provided us with all the colours that we need, to remind us of the positive words we associate with those colours as we see them in Nature; they are a gift from Nature. The more we focus on colour in Nature with the positive messages or connotations that come to us, the more balanced and in control we will feel to cope with our day-to-day problems. Being balanced using colour that comes from focusing on colour in Nature builds up our confidence and our self-worth and helps us improve our relationship with ourselves and with others.

So let us look at colour in Nature and see what messages we perceive and note the words that come to us as we imagine they would have done when humans first appeared on this Earth. In this section we give some examples of where colour in Nature occurs, and some words that come to mind as we witness and appreciate those creations.

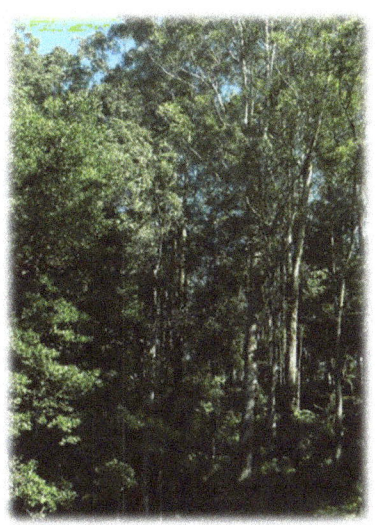

Go for a walk in a forest or park and really look at what is provided provided for us. It is *amazing*. The first thing you will notice is all all the many different shades of the colour green and then some other colours popping up here and there as well. You will notice the different *varieties* of trees and plants, and sitting under a shady tree, you will feel *protected* from the sun by the *tall* and *strong* trees that are *connected* to the land by roots that go *deep* into the earth. As you look around, you will notice you have a feeling that says *confidence* and *growth*. Some smaller trees seem to be *reaching out* for the sunlight. So, you move away from the shade of the trees to **enjoy** some sun as well and that makes you feel *warm* and *alive.* You also notice that your breathing is more *steady* as you take in the oxygen given out by the vegetation.

Then try to imagine the first humans discovering how they could make use of what would have been on offer in a forest. What there was that was edible and what was not, and what *healing* properties some plants had as well. They would have seen multi-coloured butterflies, some that are green

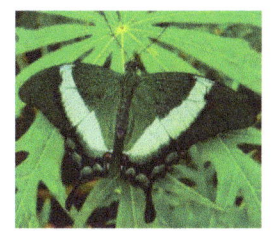

and well *camouflaged*, and they would also have noticed insects that were feeding off the vegetation. They would

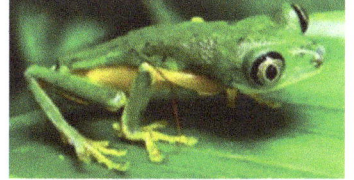

have climbed up the *tall* trees, discovered what they could see in the distance and maybe have even found birds' nests up there that were beautifully *designed*. And if there was a pond, they would have noticed some green frogs happily jumping about that made them *smile* and feel *happy.* We now know, of course, how *deserving* of our respect frogs are and so we need to take **care** of our environment because the frogs play such an *important* role in our ecology.

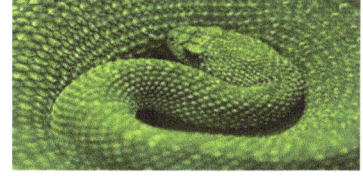

So, what is *important* in your life to focus on? Noticing a green snake cleverly *blend* in with the bushes, and the word that comes to mind might again be *camouflage* when we focus on the colour green. So, for one day perhaps try to blend in (at work or when out and about) and avoid being noticed.

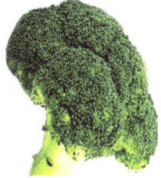

The first humans would have eaten green vegetables that they found growing that we still regard as being an important part of our diet to keep us healthy. So, we wonder how the green vegetables we now eat, such as broccoli, for instance, were *discovered* and how it came about that we now realise how many health benefits there are in what Nature provides for us. So, why not use the word *health* or *benefit.*

Think of the cucumber, for instance, so refreshing to eat. So, the words that come to mind when we think of the green coloured cucumber could be *discover, health, benefits* or *fresh*.

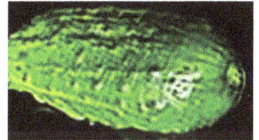

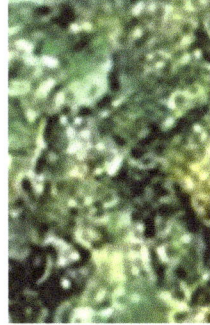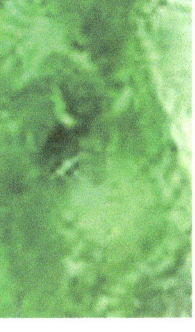

Imagine finding an *amazing* semi-*precious* green stone like the Amazonite, or the *beautiful* Tourmaline, and other *wondrous* green *precious* stones, like a green Emerald, Jade, and many others. What a *joy* that would be. How *amazing* Nature is and how many *positive* messages come to mind to make us feel *grateful* for what there is for us to *benefit* from and *enjoy* in this wonderful world we live in. And so, when we choose the colour green to focus on, we can choose any of these positive words that come to us to act upon for that day.

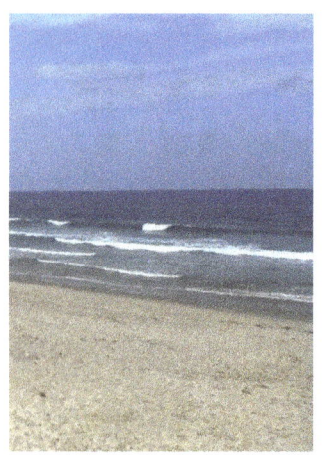

Notice, or think of, how **calm** the sea is on a **beautiful, clear** day, and the blue hue with not a cloud to be seen makes the blue in the sky more **striking**. Sitting on the sand looking out to sea makes one feel **calm** and **relaxed**. Notice the waves **constantly** coming rolling in and feel the breeze and the sun as it penetrates your skin, making you feel **warm** and **happy.** And when you **ventur**e into the water, you **appreciate** the **healthy benefit** of the sea water. Was this also how it felt for the first humans or for people from the outback who had never seen an ocean?

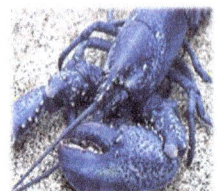

Imagine then what lies under the water, all kinds of fish, large and small; all kinds of living creatures; and corals. But there is so much more we still do not know about the sea and so it is still a **mystery.** You feel **confident** and **safe** in this wide and open space where people smile as they pass you by. No wonder people flock to the beach as often as they can. After a short, refreshing swim, walk slowly back to a shaded place while massaging your feet on the soft sand, then look back and admire such a **beautiful** sight.

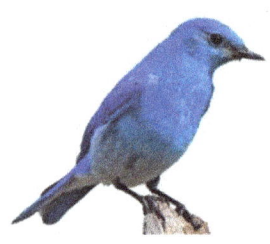

Sit in a shady spot as you look out to sea, and if you are **lucky** as you look up you may spot some blue birds that seem **happy** as they **move** about and fly from tree to tree or through some bushes to **look** for insects or honey from flowers. As they fly away, imagine where they might go and then think of all the places where you might like to go. Write them down and **imagine** going there one day. Maybe draw a blue bird, a blue butterfly, or a blue flower. How would you feel if you saw a blue butterfly for the first time?

On a drive home one day, you may see many **pretty** blue flowers growing in people's gardens or on nature strips. Perhaps play a game: spot a blue flower and see how many blue flowers you can spot in a day. Draw a blue flower or do

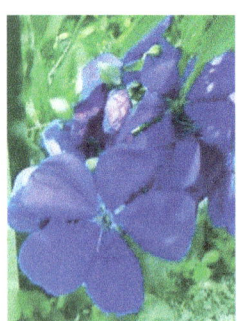

research to see how many blue flowers there are and where they might grow. Buy a blue flowering pot plant and you could even give it to someone just because you **care** to **share**. Doing this for a day will distract you from thinking negative thoughts, even if only for a while during that day and can make you feel **happy** or **uplifted**.

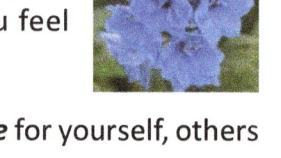

Put on a blue shirt or dress to remind yourself that if you **care** for yourself, others will **care** for you too.

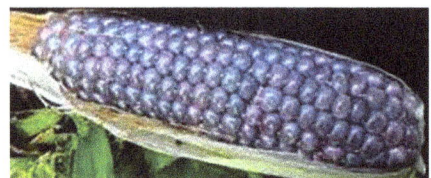

What about some fruit and vegetables that are blue? How many have you eaten, and do you have a favourite? At least **try** eating something blue, like blue corn perhaps, or some blue berries on the day you have chosen to focus on blue and the word that comes to you is **try**. Tell yourself that you will **try** something **new** that you have not tried before or have done before. Just keep those words in mind and when something **new** comes up that you have not eaten or done before, remind yourself to **try** it. It will build up your **confidence** and make you feel **proud** that you have at least given it a **try**, just for that day. These positive words or feeling will stay with you into the future.

Have you ever seen **precious** blue stones, perhaps in a ring or in a pendant? Imagine how **exciting** it would be to own such a stone. Maybe use the word **exciting** when you choose to focus on the colour blue for a day. Perhaps for that particular day, when you have chosen the colour blue and the word **exciting** to focus on you treat yourself to something you have been wanting for some time. Be **excited** that you have completed a task or project or just feel **excited** to be alive.

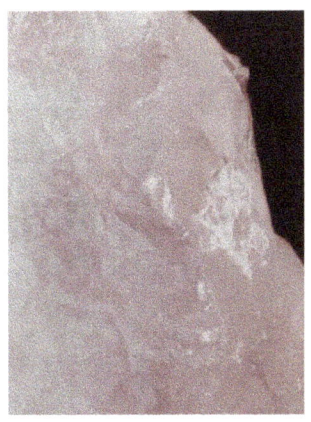

Let us look at pink in Nature. For example, think of a piece of rose quartz crystal and imagine what the first people on planet Earth would have felt if they were to suddenly **discover** a patch of **beautiful** pink colour appear where they had been digging. Imagine holding a piece of rose quartz crystal in your hands, and maybe you or the first humans, would have felt the **power** that was coming to you, and realise why pink is the colour that is often used to send messages of **love**. How **amazed** the first humans would have been to realise it was the same colour that they had seen in the sky in the late afternoon sometimes, and when the first pink buds appeared on the trees in the springtime.

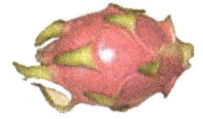

Imagine seeing a **beautiful** pink rose for the first time, and you notice that it is **delicate** and has a sweet smell that makes you feel **uplifted**. Compared to the other pink coloured flowers you may feel that you want to handle a pink rose more **gently**, just the way you would hold a new-born baby close to our chest because it is so **precious** and **fragile.** *Like a baby,* a pink rose is **soft** to the touch and has to be handled with more care. Why not buy a bunch and bring a **smile** and such **joy** *to yourself.* So, when you have chosen the colour pink for the day, it brings to mind that same feeling when you choose to focus on words like **joy, soft, delicate, fragile, sweet, gentle or feel uplifted.**

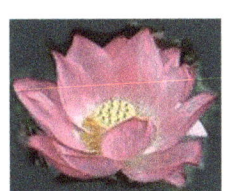

If you were to notice a pink lotus flower growing in the water of a pond what would come to your mind is that it is such an **amazing** sight of **beauty** and **purity**. And then to discover that the lotus can **regulate** its temperature similarly to the way humans do, and it can have a life span of many years. So, imagine if you are like the lotus flower and you choose either **amazing, beautiful, regulate,** or **purity**, to focus on when you choose the colour pink for the day. You may even want to draw a pink lotus flower. as you **appreciate** all that Nature has provided for us.

There are many different fruits and even vegetables that have a pink exterior or are pink on the inside. The pitaya, for instance, also known as the dragon fruit, has been discovered to have numerous **health benefits,** so focus on your **health** for a day and what can be of **benefit** to you.

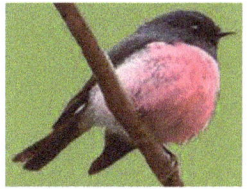

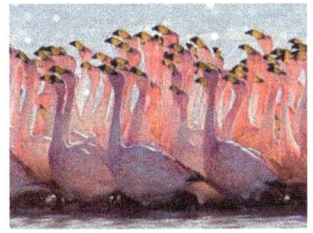

The bell jambu, like an apple, is crunchy, juicy, and **refreshing** to eat, and is so **satisfying** as well. So perhaps choose the words **refresh** or **satisfy** to focus on for the day. Maybe feel **satisfied** with your achievements or make a **fresh start** on a project.

What about all the birds that have pink feathers, like the **beautiful** Pink Robin, native to Australia? Think what other pink feathered birds there might be. Draw a picture of a pink bird and use **beautiful** to describe yourself too.

The Flamingo is a large **attractive** pink bird with a long neck, found in the shallow waters of lagoons and lakes. Flamingos live in large **social** groups and sometimes migrate to distant lands in search of small fish, insects and red algae, and other small creatures found in the muddy waters there. What words come to your mind, such as **attractive** or **social**?

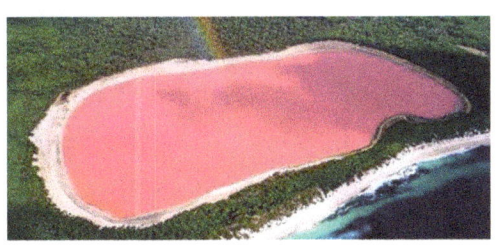

How would you feel if you came across this pink lake in Western Australia or you happen to be at the Cameron waterfalls in Canada when it turns pink because that only **rarely** happens and only in the rainy season? The words that would come to your mind would be such an **extraordinary** sight and maybe also **Wonder**, perhaps? Orwould it just be a feeling of being **curious** or **cautious** because you are not sure it is safe.

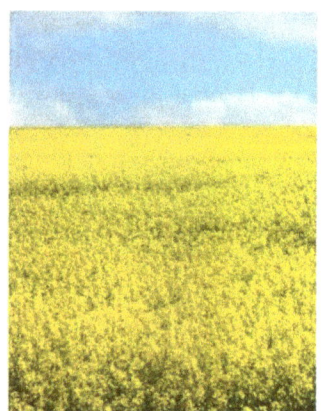

To wake up with the sunlight shining through your bedroom window and then to feel the **warmth** coming into the room, will surely make you feel **alive** and **happy**, and **ready** to **start** your day. So, **appreciate** how hard it must be for people who live in regions of the Earth where the sun does not shine for months. Imagine the first humans seeing the sun's rays **shine** through the autumn leaves of the trees. Imagine what a **pleasant** sight it must have been for our ancestors who travelled through Scotland during autumn.

Imagine if you were to drive through the countryside on a sunny morning and you suddenly came upon yellow fields that went on and on for kilometres, how would you feel? They may be fields of sunflowers or canola, which make you feel **invigorated,** and you **smile**, and feel **happy** somehow.

Imagine how it would feel to **discover** yellow gold for the first time. How **precious** that metal has became. So, choose the word **discover,** or **precious** to focus on when choosing to focus on yellow for a day.

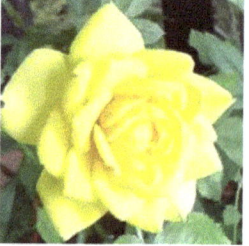

There are many fruits that are at their best when they turn yellow, meaning that they are **ripe** and **sweet** to eat: fruits like pineapples or mangoes. And not forgetting bananas and lemons as well.

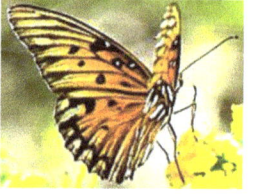

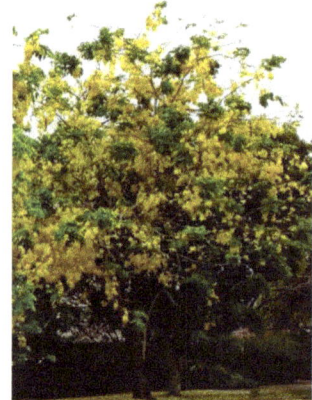

There are yellow trees, and yellow flowers, which are always such an **uplifting** sight; and, of course, the bees **love** them as much as you do.

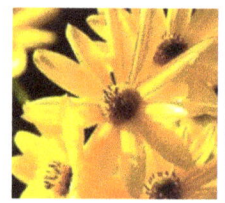

Then there are **beautiful** yellow butterflies that are so **graceful** and **silent** as they **move** from flower to flower. How short a life they have but they just do what they have to do, and no questions asked. What **beautiful** markings they have on their wings, and some are **rare** and so are **highly prized**. Imagine if we choose the colour yellow to focus on for a day and used those words: **move, highly prized, rare, beautiful,** or **graceful** to describe ourselves. We could choose **silent**, and then **silently** get on with what we have to do for that day. When we think of yellow flowers, why not take note of how the sunflower always seems to want to face where the sun comes up. How **proud** that sunflower seems. It is so **impressive** to look at.

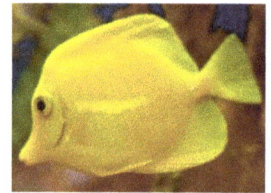

When you choose to focus on a yellow fish that is **silently** moving in a fish tank, or you **imagine** how it would if it were swimming around in the ocean? You might choose the word **imagine** and sit in the garden while imagining you are somewhere else in the world. How would that make you feel?

When you see a yellow duckling or a baby chicken that has just been born, do you think of the word **new**. These baby ducklings are also very **delicate**, so why not focus on the word **delicate**, and treat yourself **delicately** for the day? When the sun come up and a **new** day is about to **start**, can you think of something **new** that you might like to **start?**

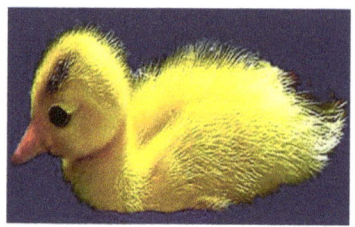

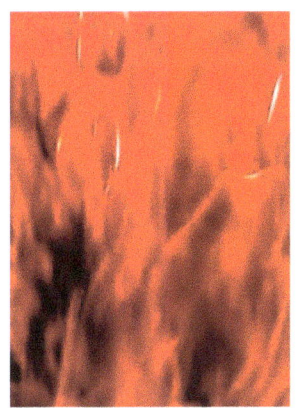

Imagine how it would have been for the first humans to see a fire that was started by lightning, roaring fiercely through a forest with no concern, it seemed, for anything in its path. Just like we would, they would certainly have been stopped in their tracks, knowing they would be at risk if they tried to **venture** forward. No wonder we use red on our **stop** signs. Only the **brave** would be fire fighters; and so red is also a colour that we associate with bravery. We, like the first humans would have been, are fascinated by fire, and there is nothing more **comforting** than sitting around a campfire or having a BBQ in the backyard; so much so, that people will often **open up** and tell stories they would normally not to **share**. We can become mesmerised looking into the flames and glowing red embers of a fire. Seeing a red sky in the late afternoon promises a **warm** day the following day, so we **prepare** for a day at the pool, or we will stay indoors with the air conditioning on! So, you may choose **venture, stop, brave, comforting, open-up, share, or warm** for the colour red.

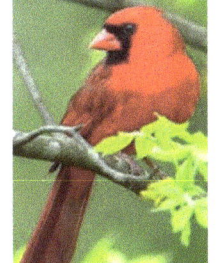

When you see a red bird what can come to your mind is, what kind of bird is that and what sound does it make and what does it eat? Just by **concentrating** on trying to spot a red bird (or on what is the coloured red in Nature) for that day will be enough to put the focus on that rather than on your worries. So, think how what is coloured red in Nature can make you feel?

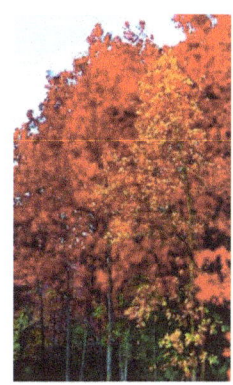

You might have noticed how some trees have leaves that **change** from green to red at certain times in the year. Or you may also have noticed trees with red flowers, like the Poinciana tree for instance, during the summer months. Look **carefully** at the **shape**, **structure** and **shades** that come from that tree. Take notice how the birds **love** to feed off the nectar.

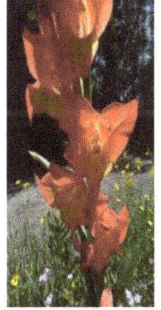

Look at gladiola flowers and notice how many **shades** of red, and **combinations** of colours, or even the **shapes**, that the flowers have. Each one is **unique** with **different** needs to make them **bloom**. What do those words mean for you **personally** when you think of your **needs** and your **uniqueness**? Hibiscus flowers that are the same colour but of all **different** shapes and sizes, are used for various traditions in many cultures. How **delicate** some flowers are and just seeing the colour red can **excite** you and you will suddenly notice other things in Nature that are also red: red fruits or vegetables, for example.

Some red berries, however, can be dangerous and is a **warning** that we should not just take anything that is red for granted so we need to take **care**. Red can remind us to be **cautious**.

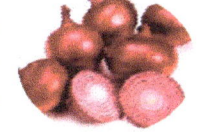

And what are the **benefits** of eating a red onion? And look how **shiny** the skin is and how many layers the onion has inside that skin. So that when choosing the colour red to focus on for a day, you might think that there are different layers to who you are or to look at what there is about life that we can study or **explore**. Meaning to look under the surface of what anything means or is about and keep on looking **deeper** into what is going on in your thoughts. Maybe put a red onion in a salad or other food you are preparing that day or **grow** some onions that day. Focusing on that task takes you away from negative thoughts even if only for a while to see that there are positives in life to think about.

Think how many **pretty, precious** stones there are that are red, and imagine how **excited** you would be to have one or a number of them set in a piece of jewellery? So, when choosing the colour red, focus on you feeling **pretty,** or that you are **precious** and what that means, or just feel **excited** about life.

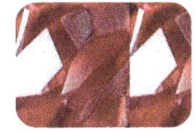

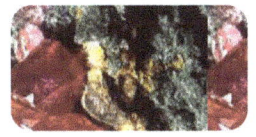
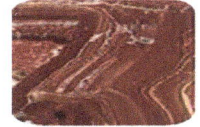
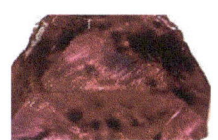

| Ruby | Red crystal rock | Onice Russo | Raw Garnet New |

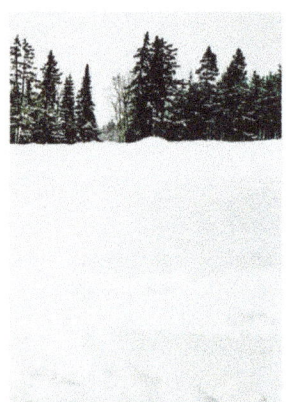

Imagine seeing the landscape blanketed in white snow, except for some green wooded areas. You can only imagine how cold it would be, and how *fresh* the air feels. You also imagine that it would be very *quiet*. The whole scene makes you feel *excited,* and it makes you feel *uplifted*. Then imagine a white Christmas and there is a colourfully decorated Christmas tree with gifts under it all wrapped in multicoloured papers and ribbons; and one of the gifts is a white canvas, some coloured paints and brushes to paint a picture to *treasure*. A *joy* forever! So why not choose the words *joy, treasure, fresh, quiet, excited,* or *uplifting* as one of the focus words when choosing the colour white for the day.

There are so many different types of white flowers and each one with its own *beauty* so that it is sometimes hard to pick a *favourite* one. Some are so tiny, some that last for such a short time, but all have an *important* role to play in our eco system. However, it is often the colour of the flower that will i**nfluence**

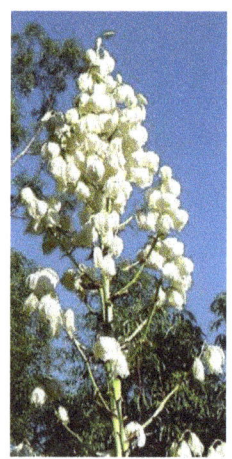

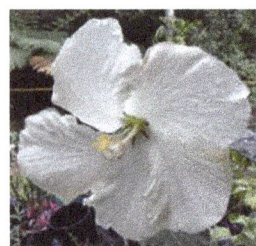

our mood and so when it is a white flower, the feeling or message that comes to us is that it is a *pure* white flower so *perfect* in *shape* and depending on the background colour of green or blue, or even if it is amongst flowers of other colours, it can still be *striking* or *stand out*. So, the words that come to mind might be *important, influence, pure, perfect, striking,* or *stand out.*

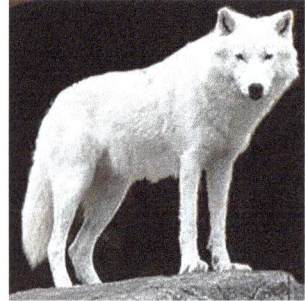

What about dogs, cats or other animals that are *pure* white. There are insects that have white skins or wings. They are all *special* and are to be *admired*. What about the *different* shades of white, when they are *comfortable*, it seems, with whatever *shade* of white they are. So, it does not matter if they are not all the same shade! We could think of the word, *special, accept, unique, shade* or *comfortable* when we choose white for the day. You could also consider some animals can *camouflage* or *blend* in when there is a need to protect themselves and just like some animals do, we can hide our true feelings. So how can you use *pure* or *different* for yourself and say how *unique* or *special* you are; what you *admire* or *accept* about yourself, when you choose one of these words to focus on the colour white.

How do you feel when you spot a *beautiful* white bird, and you just happened to have chosen to focus on white for the day? Or did you choose to focus on a white bird first and that is why you chose the colour white to focus on? Where do you look for white birds? Do you want to draw a white bird or *study* a *particular* bird, like a dove, for instance? And what about white birds that

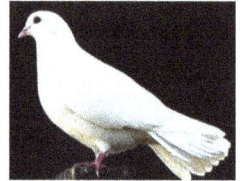

fly around the water looking for fish to eat? Just *concentrating* on trying to spot a white bird for that day will be enough to put the focus on how that colour can make you feel and how you can *expand* your *knowledge* and *appreciate* how *beautiful* Nature is.

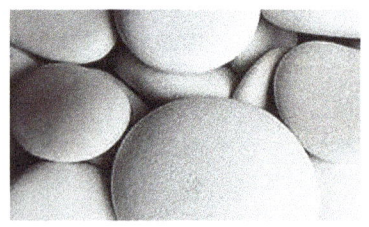

When you are looking up to see if you can spot a white bird, or birds, you can also look down and notice that there are white stones. Some white stones are *precious* gems or pearls that were started by a grain of sand entering an oyster. What thoughts come to you? Perhaps use *precious, solid, hard, shine, beautiful,* or *special* when you choose the colour white to focus on.

Wear something white and just focus on the colour white for the day to remind you of any word that the colour white in Nature brings to you. When you find it, that is then what you focus on.

Take a look at the night sky and imagine how it would be in the outback of Australia—away from the bright city lights—to experience blackness. Just as we do, the first humans would have felt that night is a time to **finish** for the day and, like them, we often feel nothing can happen until the sun comes up again the next day. As we start to **relax**, and finally we go off to our beds, **safe** in the knowledge that when we switch off the lights, we shut out the world and know for sure that no one can come into our space. As we gradually close our eyes, we **block out** everything that happened during the day; we feel we are **protected**. However, before we drift off into a deep sleep, we can hear sounds of life and wonder what or who could be roaming around in the dark. Some animals too feel **safe**, knowing that we are not there to disturb them as they are **busy** getting on with what they are there to do. And we imagine that for some couples on a **beautiful**, **cool**, starry night, with the moon shining brightly, there will be those who will walk hand-in-hand, dance the night away, or come up with a romantic song, as if they were the only ones in the world out and about on that particular dark night.

When we notice some black clouds, that often means a **warning** that a storm is about to hit us. So, we **prepare** to take shelter and wait **patiently** until the storm passes.

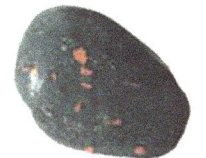

When we pick up black stones lying on the ground or by rivers and the coastline, and we notice how **solid** they are, some so smooth and shiny, there is a feeling of **wonder**. How is it that there are stones in all shapes and sizes, some *so precious*, that come out of the earth? When black opal was discovered, people were in awe and have **admired** and **treasured** opals ever since, as nothing to them is anywhere near as **precious** as a black opal. How **important** coal has been since coal was **discovered**, and charcoal too was found to be of good use. Nature has given us such **treasures** for us to use and **enjoy**, so choose one of those words that come to you.

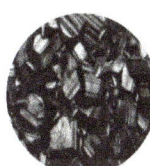

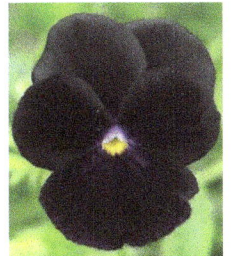

There are black flowers that certainly have their uses; some so tiny but still having a **beauty** of their own, so, use **beautiful** for your focus word.

Imagine seeing a black bear in the wild, looking so **confident, fearless,** and **strong**, or think of a black horse with its coat so **shiny** and notice how **elegant** and **strong** that horse looks. So why not have something black to wear or to have with you to remind you of those words and apply one of those words for yourself to build up your own **confidence**?

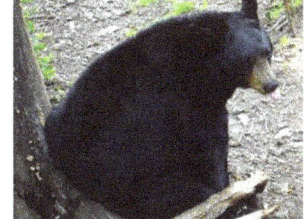

Black cats have been known to have **special** powers by some people or cultures, and so why is that? Is it the colour that makes them seem more **confident** and **mysterious** because we cannot see them at night? Is it that cats seem **proud** the way they hold their heads up and the way they move or generally how they **behave**? Imagine you having those same traits: being **mysterious** and **proud**. How would you behave when you choose the colour black, and you have chosen to focus on a black animal for the day? What characteristics do some other black animals have that you can notice and that can give you a positive word to focus on just because they are black? So, we liken the colour black to **beauty, confidence, pride, mysterious,** and **powerful**, just like when we see a **beautiful** black horse, etc. So why not take on these feeling when you choose the colour black for the day to focus on? Wear something black to remind you to focus on your chosen word for that day, or just try to notice how often you see the colour black is used and how it makes you feel in a positive way.

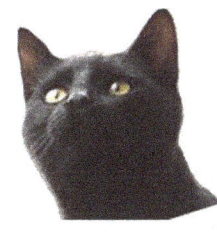

Today

Today I wake to a new day.
I know it is going to be a good day.
I see mist and morning dew,
With a sprinkling of rain.
The air so fresh and cool.
Suddenly warm, bright sunlight.
There is a gentle breeze and movements
And different smells to lift the spirit.
I hear curious different sounds
And feel the energy all around me.
There are lots of colours everywhere,
And it is such a very pleasing sight.
All that is needed for growth,
A healthy and happy life,
I feel inspired and energized.
I am so ready to get moving.
I am going to have a good day.

Adding your own choice of words

You may want to add more words that come to mind when you experience and think about the colours you see in Nature. If you truly understand the meanings of the words, you will be more empathetic with other people who use the same words you use, and you will better appreciate what Nature has to offer us. An easy way sometimes to really know the meaning of words is to make it first about someone else, and then imagine that someone is you. Ask how you feel when you discover why your friend A was looking so happy, and then imagine if A were you, how would you feel?

It might seem strange, for example, when you say that a flower is pretty and then you choose to use that word and say I am pretty when pretty can sometimes have unpleasant associations. When used as an action word, pretty could also mean that like the pretty flower, that girl is just as pleasing to look at. Meaning you are also pretty to look at. So, feel pretty and imagine you are like that flower, and you are as important as any flower or any other person. Put on a pretty dress in the chosen colour or that has that mix in it for that day to remind you to feel pretty. Another word might be discover (you might need to look up the full meaning of that word in the dictionary or to Google it). So, look for something you did not realise you could do differently. You may have told yourself that there is no way you could do a particular task, only to discover that you can do it. You may, of course, be amazed or at least feel very happy to discover that you can actually complete the task you had set for yourself that day. Write down what that task was for the day in the Action section of your Sample focus words for one week. It can be wonderful to even discover the real meaning of a word and how many ways it could be used when you look it up in a dictionary or on Google. Do not make your meditations too complicated. Keep them light and easy but as deep and meaningful as you wish. We live mostly in our imagination and imagine things that sometimes are not true or will never happen. We imagine what our day will be like and then make it a reality. But good or bad, it is up to ourselves to bring our thinking into balance. So, imagine you want to focus on one particular idea that comes to mind. Each day is different and, for example, when choosing the colour yellow to focus on perhaps the first thing that comes to your mind is a huge, delicious, sweet ripe, yellow mango. You might see yourself going to a supermarket and looking at a display of mangoes; you feel excited and choose the best one there; you think how you will prepare it when you get home; your mouth is watering as you see yourself slicing the mango and you can actually taste it; you then think how far that mango has travelled to now be in your hands; see a tree full of mangoes, maybe in an orchard; the people who had to pick and pack those mangoes; and you think about the farmer who grew them and nurtured those mango trees; the early humans who first discovered that that fruit was safe to eat. You will never again take a mango for granted because you feel lucky that it has been made available for to you to enjoy. You may wear something in yellow and see what else you can see in yellow from Nature that is all around you. Or you may wish to just draw or paint a picture of a bowl of fruit and make a mango the main feature; or you might even like to write a poem.

Here is a sample of some wise words for the colour red:

A Bowl of Tomatoes

A bowl of tomatoes, a picture of delight I would like to share with you. Red, yellow, or black, and so juicy, just one will satisfy me and I am sure you will think so too. So many options, but eaten fresh just picked, with a sprinkling of salt will do nicely. Tomato soup, my next favourite, and is a pizza without tomato a pizza? To see them grow in my garden, I sure can't wait for them to ripen, but it's a race with the insects, who like them just as much as I do. So, appreciate the tomato next time you have one, and all the other fruits and veggies too, but also appreciate the people who grow them and share them with us; farmers who work on the land so we can continue living in the city. Next time you pick up a piece of fruit or some veggies in your shop, smile and be grateful that the farmers are thinking of us, and always try to produce the best crop they can, no matter what challenges they have to face.

If we do this with everything that Nature has provided for us all, and especially with our fellow humans, then would we not take more care of what we have? Be more open to trying a different word each day, because if we know and have experienced how it felt when using the different words? It makes us more empathetic. The best way to start is with the list of words provided in the order they have been listed to ensure you use and experience each word yourself. You can always add more positive words based on your own further experiences with Nature. The order of the chosen colour is up to the individual but as long as that colour and word are not repeated two days running. You may also decide to start your week on a Monday, but do not have the same colour every Monday. Whenever you think of more words you want to add, write them down, so you will remember them and can use them as you need to. You may even want to express yourself in a different language. Balance With Colour (or BWC) does not have any hard and fast rules to follow, except for not using the same colour or the word on two consecutive days, because the more different words you use the more empathetic you will be, and that is a win-win for all. The more you use the Balance With Colour technique the easier and more natural it will become for you to avoid the negativity and the scaremongering we hear almost every day. Consequently, the more we appreciate how Nature works.

More Sample Focus Words

Here are some quick reference words you might associate with each of the seven colours. Remember to first choose where you see what is in your chosen colour in Nature and then notice the word that comes to mind. That chosen word will have to fit in not matter what happens on that day.

Green

Variety, Positive, Grateful, Stand tall, Pride, Outdoor, Relaxation, Feeling uplifted, Cool, Abundance, Appreciate, Steady, Hopeful, Treat, Harmony, Self-worth, Deserving, Adaptable, Feel alive, Peaceful, Tolerant, Patience, Sharing, Useful, Working together, Calm, Change...

Blue

Peaceful, Fresh, Healing, Warning, Future, Expansive, Fun, Ambition, Hopeful, Optimistic, Adaptable, Careful, Abundance, Anticipate, Refresh, Trust, Honesty, Protected, Truth, Order, Safe, Clear, Striking, Constantly, Cool...

Pink

Gently, Start, Kind, Loving, Calm, Nurturing, Warm, New, Power, Amazing, Fragile, Health, harmony, Refreshing...

Yellow

Brightness, Joy, Uplifting, Alert, Light, Cheerful, Energetic, Healthy. Optimistic, Invigorate, Smile, Ripe, Sweet, Love, Beautiful, Graceful, Silent, Proud...

Red

Unique, Heat, Energy, Motivation, Active, Passionate, Courageous, Action, Strong, Fearless, Delicate, Moving forward, Fired up, Game, Prepare, Concentrating, Change, Carefully, Fast, Warning, Beautiful, Need, Love, Excited, Different...

White

Cool, Soft, Blank, Surprise, Holiness, New, Starting, Fresh, Beginning, Influence, Awake, New idea, Open, Optimistic, Wonder, Trustworthy, Important, Excited, Uplifted, Treasure, Joy, Pure, Quiet, Peace, Shades...

Black

Stop, Silent, Hide, Private, In awe, Shine, Closure, Dream, Focus, Close eyes, Beautiful, Protected, Warning, Prepare, Smooth, Shiny, Communicate, More, Direction, ...

Sample words associated with each of the seven colours

When you choose the colour **pink** and you see, or imagine seeing, a beautiful **pink** rose in your garden, think of the word *beautiful* or how *delicate* it is. And so, focus on one of those words. You might even notice other **pink** flowers in your garden and say how *lucky* you are to have such *beautiful* flowers there. So, every time you notice the colour **pink,** remind yourself to focus on either the word *beautiful, delicate* or *lucky* to lift your spirits for the day. Think how you have to *care* for your **pink** flowers and do the same for yourself.

The following day, choose the colour **blue** and think of the ocean and how you would feel if you went for a swim that day. Maybe even go to a beach and choose *fresh, healing, or relaxing* to focus on for the whole day. Make it about you, so you might think of making a *fresh* start on something or to put on *relaxing* music for that day.

Choose **black** the next day and imagine what it would feel like to look at a **black** stone. It might be any kind of **black** stone even a stone you see around your garden that is *solid, smooth,* and *shiny* so you could decide to be *solid* in any commitment you have made or are about to make or be sure everything runs *smoothly,* so be more prepared. Or you could just remind yourself to notice everything that is *shiny*. Perhaps pick up and carry a **black** stone with you to remind yourself to focus on those words.

On the fourth day, choose to focus on the colour **yellow**, and imagine being in the middle of a field full of sunflowers, and you feel really *happy.* Wear something **yellow** or just draw a sunflower with a *smiling* face in the middle. Every time you see the colour **yellow**, say the word *happy* and *smile*. That will lifts your spirits for the whole day and surely will have a flow-on effect to others making it a win-win for all.

For the fifth day, you might look up at the sky first thing in the morning and notice quite a few **white** clouds about and that they are *moving fast* across the sky as if in a *hurry* to get somewhere *important*. What if you decide to make a *move just like the moving* clouds because you have goals you need to achieve, and they are *important* to you. Or you could focus on the colour **white** itself and wear something in **white** for the day.

Choosing **red** for the second last day of your *Balance With Colour* activity, so why not just focus on the colour **red** in nature for the day. The words that then come to mind is *Appreciate* what a *beautiful* colour **red** is and that it is a gift from nature that makes you feel *uplifted*. You might even notice that colour in a picture or count how many things are of a **red** colour in your home. You may like to wear something that is coloured **red,** eat a **red** tomato or make a **red** jelly.

Choose **green** on the last day of your *Balance With Colour* activity for the week. You then happen to look out of your window at a tree in front of your house, and you wonder how tall it will eventually *grow*. So, you decide to focus on the word *grow*, and wonder how can you *grow*? *Grow* your business or *grow* in *confidence for that day*. Keep thinking about it and you will be sure to come up with an idea. And if you do not, at least you can put your focus on the colour **green** or on the tree and that can distract you from thinking negatively.

How the *Balance With Colour* works

Most people do their journaling at night to reflect on the day just passed. In the *Balance With Colour* Journal, we focus on our intent for the day ahead. We choose a colour in Nature, study something in Nature that is of that colour, then choose our word from those that come to mind as we realise what Nature is telling us. We then look up the meaning of that word so that we can use that word for our positive action to balance out any negative thoughts or events the next day. The best time to do this is at the end of the day, so that we have our purpose for the next day in mind first thing in the morning. At the end of the day we reflect and record how we felt about having used that intent. Another way is to choose your colour the night before but leave the intent for the next day while doing your BWC Meditation. When you are ready and you have decided on the word you want to focus on for that day, record the word you have chosen in your journal and also the meaning of that word, as shown in the Sample Focus Words page provided. At the end of the day, write how you felt about your positive action for that day, so that you can add more positive words to your vocabulary.

Bad happens and it is up to us ourselves to not make it worse than what it already is by having negative thoughts that are sometimes only just in our imagination. So, why not focus on solving whatever the problem may be in a positive and balanced way or to distract yourself even for a short time. Sharing the *Balance With Colour* Journal with family is a great way for bonding and learning. It is educational and fun, while at the same time it can make us appreciate what is fascinating about our world when we appreciate what Nature has provided for us. Colour is all around, and it can lift our spirits

In our so often busy, busy lifestyle, we might not have time to do any routine exercise or to meditate, which also involves being conscious of our breathing. So, the best way to start the day off is to set the alarm five to ten minutes early (or longer if you wish) so you have the extra time for our recommended morning exercise while still lying in bed. Remove your pillow and, just like all babies do when they wake up normally, stretch your whole body and roll over left to right in any way you feel comfortable to do so. Stretch out and bend your arms and your legs in any direction that suits you and is comfortable to do. Rotate your hands and feet and wriggle your fingers and toes. Next, slowly turn your head from side to side, down and up a number of times. Then stretch your mouth wide open as if you are yawning, you can even make a noise and make some funny faces. Squeeze your lips together this way and that way and finish with a smile. Slowly blink your eyes open and closed while giving them a squeeze and repeat it as you feel the need. Holding your head still, move your eyes to the left and right, up and down, and round and round, and repeat that a few times. Finally, cross your arms over to massage and squeeze both your arms right down to your hands and fingers; then massage your body, your face and the top of your head. Cross your legs and run one leg over the other, and with your feet rub, your legs and feet. The next step is to close your eyes again and to the count of four, take a slow deep breath in, and then breathe out to the count of five. Do that as many times as you like.

Finally, do your *Balance With Colour* Meditation: relax and try to visualise where you might see the colour you have chosen the night before in as many natural settings as you can (some samples are given in the Colour in Nature section in this book, or you can find them on Google). When you are satisfied, and you feel ready to get up and start your day, you have that colour and word to focus on. You can even do more exercises or other types of meditation if that is your normal routine to do so.

If you have not done the Balance With Colour routine or the exercise we have recommend, do not worry because you can still do it the next day or some other time that is more convenient for you. However, the more you practice Balance With Colour, the more it will become second nature. You may even want to change some of what we have recommended, or you already have your own way of starting your day. The main thing is to start your day on a positive note and look forward to a new day.

During the day, remember to use the positive word you have chosen as many times as you can or feel the need to do so. And if you feel overwhelmed, tense or even a little depressed, because we all can suddenly feel that way sometimes for some reason during the day, or it could be just the weather, just close your eyes for a few minutes to do a quick meditation on your focus for the day while doing some gentle breathing exercises. We often forget how important our breathing is especially when we are tense, so it is a good idea to focus on our breathing while focusing on our chosen colour and where in Nature we see that colour. There are many different methods of breathing, and you may already have chosen the one you feel comfortable with. However, we recommend Dr. Doe Lang's method to use during the day when you need to focus on your breathing to feel calm. For instance, when there is a stressful situation happening or you just need a burst of energy. using your thumb and fore finger on your right hand, close your left nostril with your fore finger and breathe in through the right nostril. Then close that right nostril with your thumb and open the left side to breathe out through your left nostril. Repeat a number of times, and then using your left hand, do the same. This breathing exercise can be done very discreetly anytime anywhere, if you do not want to draw attention to the fact that you are stressed or are focusing on your breathing.

Finally, when you are ready to go to sleep, relax and do some slow deep breathing exercise. Repeat a few times and you will be sure to have a sound sleep. If you do wake up during the night repeat your breathing exercise and focus on your positive intentions or how wonderful and interesting Nature is. *Balance With Colour* can help you do that.

Sample focus sheet for one week

With space for date and Notes as a reminder for that day (e.g., birthdays, appointments etc)

(1/1) *Notes:* NEW YEAR: *A day to relax and go to the beach with family....*

Colour: **GREEN**

Word: *Grow (having noticed how a particular tree in my garden has grown)*

Meaning: *Expand and or add to an idea.*

Action: *I decided to focus on putting more of the ideas I have into my writing today so that I can share those ideas with more people.*

How I felt: *It was exciting because I came up with even more ideas to add to my writing.*

===

(2/1) *Notes:* *Go shopping...*

Colour: **WHITE**

Word: *Pure (I was imagining seeing water in a stream that had no contamination)*

Meaning: *Meaning it has no blemishes or is unmixed with other matter*

Action: *I decided that I would not eat or drink anything with added flavour or preservatives, and only drink plain water for today.*

How I felt: *I appreciated how Nature had intended us to taste things as they are meant to be.*

===

(   ) *Notes:*

Colour: **RED**

Word: *Stop (stop and think about how hot the chilli is that I have chosen)*

Meaning: *Pause for a second and think about what to do or say*

Action: *I reminded myself to stop and think first every time I wanted to say something or answer a question to make sure I gave the right information or impression.*

How I felt: *It made me felt more confident and surer of myself.*

===

(   ) *Notes:*

Colour: **BLUE**

Word: *Calm (imagine sitting at the beach and seeing how calm the sea is)*

Meaning: *Not get upset or react too hastily.*

Action: *I will tell myself to take a deep breath and stay calm if I feel something getting stressful anytime today. Count to ten before reacting.*

How I felt: *I felt calm and in control when I had a couple of stressful situations.*

===

(   ) *Notes:*

Colour: **BLACK**

Word: *Silent (observing the stillness of the night when everything is silent)*

Meaning: *To not make a sound*

Action: *I decided I would silently get on with my work today and did not talk about anything that was not important.*

How I felt: *I was amazed at how much work I got done because I used my time wisely.*

===

(   ) *Notes:*

Colour: **YELLOW**

Word: *Bright (seeing yellow flowers that brightens up the garden)*

Meaning: *Being striking and can light up or catch your eyes*

Action: *I wore a yellow shirt and focused on the colour yellow, especially in the garden. It was amazing how many yellow flowers I noticed were now growing there.*

How I felt: *It lifted my spirits and made me feel happy whenever I thought about it.*

===

(   ) *Notes:*

Colour: **PINK**

Word: *Beautiful (thinking of pink rose quartz crystal)*

Meaning: *Meaning pleasing to the senses and the mind*

Action: *I wore a beautiful pink bracelet that my friend Skye had given me to remind me to look at and to appreciate the beauty in all that Nature has created*

How I felt: *I realise that I can see beauty everywhere if I set my mind to think that way.*

===

Sample Summary/Intention page

The Summary/Intention *page is there to record in more detail what is experienced after each four-week period. Remembering to also make sure you put the date when you started on the top of the page. The Summary/Intention page is important for when you want to take stock and reflect on the progress you are making. To record how you were able to handle stressful situations by having colour to remind you of the positive word you had chosen to focus on for a particular stressful situation, or to write in more detail some interesting findings you may have learned or experienced. This is important if you want to quickly see the progress you are making.*

There is also a Final Summary at the end of the year to reflect on how your year has been: write a story about your achievements; or your adventure; paste a photo or two; add a poem; wise saying; make up a mantra to use daily if you wish; etc. And finally add important phone numbers and other reference information on the last page.

As for your intention, did you specifically think of something about yourself that you wanted to change in some way? In other words, did you consciously think how you may come across to other people? We all have good intentions and goals, but do we even remember them? Do we get distracted and then feel disappointed that we did not achieve them? Write down your goals and when you hope to achieve them and make notes of how you are progressing towards those goals. That can help to spur you on and get you excited and happy to see what you have accomplished. You might say, I want to stop being judgmental. So, write down if you noticed when you have avoided being judgemental. That way you will become more conscious of this character flaw and gradually you will stop doing it. You have been told that you speak too loudly. So, are you speaking more softly now? Did you complete a task you have been working on that was overdue? Did you do some jobs that you have been meaning to do but have procrastinated? You promised to do regular exercise. Are you exercising regularly?

Here are some questions that you may also ask yourself:
Do I look to colour in Nature for more inspiration?
Do I wear something in the colour I chose for the day?
Do I notice the colour I chose for that day everywhere I looked?
Have I noticed that I am now more in control of my moods?
Am I using more positive words?
Have I shared the *Balance With Colour* technique with someone?
Do I feel more comfortable to do the *Balance With Colour* technique privately?
Do I find doing the *Balance With Colour* technique fun and easy to use?
Did I discover different ways to use the *Balance With Colour* technique?

These are questions and some ideas for you to consider and to keep you on track with your positive intention and for it to become a habit. If you stick to your intention, you will feel proud of yourself.

Balance With Colour it is about your personal development. You cannot change other people, but you can feel a lot happier if you achieve what you set out to do or you know you need to do that. However, you may already see a change after one or two weeks. The more often you apply the Balance With Colour technique, the more it will come naturally to you to think positively and appreciate Nature.

Focus words week 1 (Date   )

(   ) *Notes:*
Colour: GREEN
Word:
Meaning:
Action:

How I felt:

===

(   ) *Notes:*
Colour: WHITE
Word:
Meaning:
Action:

How I felt:

===

(   ) *Notes:*
Colour: RED
Word:
Meaning:
Action:

How I felt:

===

(   ) *Notes:*
Colour: BLUE
Word:
Meaning:
Action:

How I felt:

===

(   ) *Notes:*
Colour: BLACK
Word:
Meaning:
Action:

How I felt:

===

(   ) *Notes:*
Colour: YELLOW
Word:
Meaning:
Action:

How I felt:

===

(   ) *Notes:*
Colour: PINK
Word:
Meaning:
Action:

How I felt:

===

Focus words for week 2 (Date   )

(   ) *Notes:*
Colour: **GREEN**
Word:
Meaning:
Action:

How I felt:
==

(   ) *Notes:*
Colour: **WHITE**
Word:
Meaning:
Action:

How I felt:
==

(   ) *Notes:*
Colour: **RED**
Word:
Meaning:
Action:

How I felt:
==

(   ) *Notes:*
Colour: **BLUE**
Word:
Meaning:
Action:

How I felt:
==

(   ) *Notes:*
Colour: **BLACK**
Word:
Meaning:
Action:

How I felt:
==

(   ) *Notes:*
Colour: **YELLOW**
Word:
Meaning:
Action:

How I felt:
==

(   ) *Notes:*
Colour: **PINK**
Word:
Meaning:
Action:

How I felt:
==

(   ) *Notes:*
Colour: **GREEN**
Word:
Meaning:
Action:

How I felt:
===

(   ) *Notes:*
Colour: **WHITE**
Word:
Meaning:
Action:

How I felt:
===

(   ) *Notes:*
Colour: **RED**
Word:
Meaning:
Action:

How I felt:
===

(   ) *Notes:*
Colour: **BLUE**
Word:
Meaning:
Action:

How I felt:
===

(   ) *Notes:*
Colour: **BLACK**
Word:
Meaning:
Action:

How I felt:
===

(   ) *Notes:*
Colour: **YELLOW**
Word:
Meaning:
Action:

How I felt:
===

(   ) *Notes:*
Colour: **PINK**
Word:
Meaning:
Action:

How I felt:
===

Focus words for week 4 (Date   )

(   ) *Notes:*
Colour: **GREEN**
Word:
Meaning:
Action:

How I felt:
===

(   ) *Notes:*
Colour: **WHITE**
Word:
Meaning:
Action:

How I felt:
===

(   ) *Notes:*
Colour: **RED**
Word:
Meaning:
Action:

How I felt:
===

(   ) *Notes:*
Colour: **BLUE**
Word:
Meaning:
Action:

How I felt:
===

(   ) *Notes:*
Colour: **BLACK**
Word:
Meaning:
Action:

How I felt:
===

(   ) *Notes:*
Colour: **YELLOW**
Word:
Meaning:
Action:

How I felt:
===

(   ) *Notes:*
Colour: **PINK**
Word:
Meaning:
Action:

How I felt:
===

Summary/Intention (Date   )

(   ) *Notes:*
Colour: | WHITE |
Word:
Meaning:
Action:

How I felt:
===

(   ) *Notes:*
Colour: | BLUE |
Word:
Meaning:
Action:

How I felt:
===

(   ) *Notes:*
Colour: | PINK |
Word:
Meaning:
Action:

How I felt:
===

(   ) *Notes:*
Colour: | YELLOW |
Word:
Meaning:
Action:

How I felt:
===

(   ) *Notes:*
Colour: | RED |
Word:
Meaning:
Action:

How I felt:
===

(   ) *Notes:*
Colour: | GREEN |
Word:
Meaning:
Action:

How I felt:
===

(   ) *Notes:*
Colour: | BLACK |
Word:
Meaning:
Action:

How I felt:
===

Focus words for week 6 (Date   )

(   ) *Notes:*
Colour: **WHITE**
Word:
Meaning:
Action:

How I felt:
===

(   ) *Notes:*
Colour: **BLUE**
Word:
Meaning:
Action:

How I felt:
===

(   ) *Notes:*
Colour: **PINK**
Word:
Meaning:
Action:

How I felt:
===

(   ) *Notes:*
Colour: **YELLOW**
Word:
Meaning:
Action:

How I felt:
===

(   ) *Notes:*
Colour: **RED**
Word:
Meaning:
Action:

How I felt:
===

(   ) *Notes:*
Colour: **GREEN**
Word:
Meaning:
Action:

How I felt:
===

(   ) *Notes:*
Colour: **BLACK**
Word:
Meaning:
Action:

How I felt:
===

Focus words for week 7 (Date   )

(   ) *Notes:*
Colour: `WHITE`
Word:
Meaning:
Action:

How I felt:
===

(   ) *Notes:*
Colour: `BLUE`
Word:
Meaning:
Action:

How I felt:
===

(   ) *Notes:*
Colour: `PINK`
Word:
Meaning:
Action:

How I felt:
===

(   ) *Notes:*
Colour: `YELLOW`
Word:
Meaning:
Action:

How I felt:
===

(   ) *Notes:*
Colour: `RED`
Word:
Meaning:
Action:

How I felt:
===

(   ) *Notes:*
Colour: `GREEN`
Word:
Meaning:
Action:

How I felt:
===

(   ) *Notes:*
Colour: `BLACK`
Word:
Meaning:
Action:

How I felt:
===

(   ) *Notes:*

Colour: WHITE

Word:

Meaning:

Action:

How I felt:

===

(   ) *Notes:*

Colour: BLUE

Word:

Meaning:

Action:

How I felt:

===

(   ) *Notes:*

Colour: PINK

Word:

Meaning:

Action:

How I felt:

===

(   ) *Notes:*

Colour: YELLOW

Word:

Meaning:

Action:

How I felt:

===

(   ) *Notes:*

Colour: RED

Word:

Meaning:

Action:

How I felt:

===

(   ) *Notes:*

Colour: GREEN

Word:

Meaning:

Action:

How I felt:

===

(   ) *Notes:*

Colour: BLACK

Word:

Meaning:

Action:

How I felt:

===

Summary/Intention (week 9-12)

Focus words for week 9 (Date   )

(   ) *Notes:*
Colour: **BLUE**
Word:
Meaning:
Action:

How I felt:
==

(   ) *Notes:*
Colour: **GREEN**
Word:
Meaning:
Action:

How I felt:
==

(   ) *Notes:*
Colour: **WHITE**
Word:
Meaning:
Action:

How I felt:
==

(   ) *Notes:*
Colour: **RED**
Word:
Meaning:
Action:

How I felt:
==

(   ) *Notes:*
Colour: **BLACK**
Word:
Meaning:
Action:

How I felt:
==

(   ) *Notes:*
Colour: **YELLOW**
Word:
Meaning:
Action:

How I felt:
==

(   ) *Notes:*
Colour: **PINK**
Word:
Meaning:
Action:

How I felt:
==

Focus words for week 10 (Date   )

(   ) *Notes:*
Colour: BLUE
Word:
Meaning:
Action:

How I felt:
===

(   ) *Notes:*
Colour: GREEN
Word:
Meaning:
Action:

How I felt:
===

(   ) *Notes:*
Colour: WHITE
Word:
Meaning:
Action:

How I felt:
===

(   ) *Notes:*
Colour: RED
Word:
Meaning:
Action:

How I felt:
===

(   ) *Notes:*
Colour: BLACK
Word:
Meaning:
Action:

How I felt:
===

(   ) *Notes:*
Colour: YELLOW
Word:
Meaning:
Action:

How I felt:
===

(   ) *Notes:*
Colour: PINK
Word:
Meaning:
Action:

How I felt:
===

Focus words for week 11 (Date   )

(   ) *Notes:*
Colour: **BLUE**
Word:
Meaning:
Action:

How I felt:
===

(   ) *Notes:*
Colour: **GREEN**
Word:
Meaning:
Action:

How I felt:
===

(   ) *Notes:*
Colour: **WHITE**
Word:
Meaning:
Action:

How I felt:
===

(   ) *Notes:*
Colour: **RED**
Word:
Meaning:
Action:

How I felt:
===

(   ) *Notes:*
Colour: **BLACK**
Word:
Meaning:
Action:

How I felt:
===

(   ) *Notes:*
Colour: **YELLOW**
Word:
Meaning:
Action:

How I felt:
===

(   ) *Notes:*
Colour: **PINK**
Word:
Meaning:
Action:

How I felt:
===

(   ) *Notes:*
Colour: BLUE
Word:
Meaning:
Action:

How I felt:
===
(   ) *Notes:*
Colour: GREEN
Word:
Meaning:
Action:

How I felt:
===
(   ) *Notes:*
Colour: WHITE
Word:
Meaning:
Action:

How I felt:
===
(   ) *Notes:*
Colour: RED
Word:
Meaning:
Action:

How I felt:
===
(   ) *Notes:*
Colour: BLACK
Word:
Meaning:
Action:

How I felt:
===
(   ) *Notes:*
Colour: YELLOW
Word:
Meaning:
Action:

How I felt:
===
(   ) *Notes:*
Colour: PINK
Word:
Meaning:
Action:

How I felt:
===

Summary/Intention (Date   )

Focus words for week 13 (Date   )

( ) *Notes:*
Colour: **BLACK**
Word:
Meaning:
Action:

How I felt:
===

( ) *Notes:*
Colour: **GREEN**
Word:
Meaning:
Action:

How I felt:
===

( ) *Notes:*
Colour: **WHITE**
Word:
Meaning:
Action:

How I felt:
===

( ) *Notes:*
Colour: **RED**
Word:
Meaning:
Action:

How I felt:
===

( ) *Notes:*
Colour: **PINK**
Word:
Meaning:
Action:

How I felt:
===

( ) *Notes:*
Colour: **YELLOW**
Word:
Meaning:
Action:

How I felt:
===

( ) *Notes:*
Colour: **BLUE**
Word:
Meaning:
Action:

How I felt:
===

Focus words for week 14 (Date   )

(   ) *Notes:*
Colour: **BLACK**
Word:
Meaning:
Action:

How I felt:
===

(   ) *Notes:*
Colour: **GREEN**
Word:
Meaning:
Action:

How I felt:
===

(   ) *Notes:*
Colour: **WHITE**
Word:
Meaning:
Action:

How I felt:
===

(   ) *Notes:*
Colour: **RED**
Word:
Meaning:
Action:

How I felt:
===

(   ) *Notes:*
Colour: **PINK**
Word:
Meaning:
Action:

How I felt:
===

(   ) *Notes:*
Colour: **YELLOW**
Word:
Meaning:
Action:

How I felt:
===

(   ) *Notes:*
Colour: **BLUE**
Word:
Meaning:
Action:

How I felt:
===

Focus words for week 15 (Date   )

(   ) *Notes:*
Colour: **BLACK**
Word:
Meaning:
Action:

How I felt:
===

(   ) *Notes:*
Colour: **GREEN**
Word:
Meaning:
Action:

How I felt:
===

(   ) *Notes:*
Colour: **WHITE**
Word:
Meaning:
Action:

How I felt:
===

(   ) *Notes:*
Colour: **RED**
Word:
Meaning:
Action:

How I felt:
===

(   ) *Notes:*
Colour: **PINK**
Word:
Meaning:
Action:

How I felt:
===

(   ) *Notes:*
Colour: **YELLOW**
Word:
Meaning:
Action:

How I felt:
===

(   ) *Notes:*
Colour: **BLUE**
Word:
Meaning:
Action:

How I felt:
===

Focus words for week 16 (Date   )

(   ) *Notes:*
Colour: **BLACK**
Word:
Meaning:
Action:

How I felt:

===

(   ) *Notes:*
Colour: **GREEN**
Word:
Meaning:
Action:

How I felt:

===

(   ) *Notes:*
Colour: **WHITE**
Word:
Meaning:
Action:

How I felt:

===

(   ) *Notes:*
Colour: **RED**
Word:
Meaning:
Action:

How I felt:

===

(   ) *Notes:*
Colour: **PINK**
Word:
Meaning:
Action:

How I felt:

===

(   ) *Notes:*
Colour: **YELLOW**
Word:
Meaning:
Action:

How I felt:

===

(   ) *Notes:*
Colour: **BLUE**
Word:
Meaning:
Action:

How I felt:

===

Summary/Intention (Date   )

Focus words for week 17 (Date   )

(   ) *Notes:*
Colour: **RED**
Word:
Meaning:
Action:

How I felt:
===

(   ) *Notes:*
Colour: **BLACK**
Word:
Meaning:
Action:

How I felt:
===

(   ) *Notes:*
Colour: **BLUE**
Word:
Meaning:
Action:

How I felt:
===

(   ) *Notes:*
Colour: **YELLOW**
Word:
Meaning:
Action:

How I felt:
===

(   ) *Notes:*
Colour: **PINK**
Word:
Meaning:
Action:

How I felt:
===

(   ) *Notes:*
Colour: **GREEN**
Word:
Meaning:
Action:

How I felt:
===

(   ) *Notes:*
Colour: **WHITE**
Word:
Meaning:
Action:

How I felt:
===

Focus words for week 18 (Date   )

(   ) *Notes:*
Colour: **RED**
Word:
Meaning:
Action:

How I felt:
===

(   ) *Notes:*
Colour: **BLACK**
Word:
Meaning:
Action:

How I felt:
===

(   ) *Notes:*
Colour: **BLUE**
Word:
Meaning:
Action:

How I felt:
===

(   ) *Notes:*
Colour: **YELLOW**
Word:
Meaning:
Action:

How I felt:
===

(   ) *Notes:*
Colour: **PINK**
Word:
Meaning:
Action:

How I felt:
===

(   ) *Notes:*
Colour: **GREEN**
Word:
Meaning:
Action:

How I felt:
===

(   ) *Notes:*
Colour: **WHITE**
Word:
Meaning:
Action:

How I felt:
===

(   ) *Notes:*

Colour: RED

Word:

Meaning:

Action:

How I felt:

==

(   ) *Notes:*

Colour: BLACK

Word:

Meaning:

Action:

How I felt:

==

(   ) *Notes:*

Colour: BLUE

Word:

Meaning:

Action:

How I felt:

==

(   ) *Notes:*

Colour: YELLOW

Word:

Meaning:

Action:

How I felt:

==

(   ) *Notes:*

Colour: PINK

Word:

Meaning:

Action:

How I felt:

==

(   ) *Notes:*

Colour: GREEN

Word:

Meaning:

Action:

How I felt:

==

(   ) *Notes:*

Colour: WHITE

Word:

Meaning:

Action:

How I felt:

==

Focus words for week 20 (Date   )

(   ) *Notes:*
Colour: **RED**
Word:
Meaning:
Action:

How I felt:

===

(   ) *Notes:*
Colour: **BLACK**
Word:
Meaning:
Action:

How I felt:

===

(   ) *Notes:*
Colour: **BLUE**
Word:
Meaning:
Action:

How I felt:

===

(   ) *Notes:*
Colour: **YELLOW**
Word:
Meaning:
Action:

How I felt:

===

(   ) *Notes:*
Colour: **PINK**
Word:
Meaning:
Action:

How I felt:

===

(   ) *Notes:*
Colour: **GREEN**
Word:
Meaning:
Action:

How I felt:

===

(   ) *Notes:*
Colour: **WHITE**
Word:
Meaning:
Action:

How I felt:

===

Summary/Intention (Date   )

Focus words for week 21 (Date   )

(   ) *Notes:*
Colour: **YELLOW**
Word:
Meaning:
Action:

How I felt:
===

(   ) *Notes:*
Colour: **GREEN**
Word:
Meaning:
Action:

How I felt:
===

(   ) *Notes:*
Colour: **WHITE**
Word:
Meaning:
Action:

How I felt:
===

(   ) *Notes:*
Colour: **PINK**
Word:
Meaning:
Action:

How I felt:
===

(   ) *Notes:*
Colour: **BLUE**
Word:
Meaning:
Action:

How I felt:
===

(   ) *Notes:*
Colour: **BLACK**
Word:
Meaning:
Action:

How I felt:
===

(   ) *Notes:*
Colour: **RED**
Word:
Meaning:
Action:

How I felt:
===

Focus words for week 22 (Date   )

(   ) *Notes:*
Colour: **YELLOW**
Word:
Meaning:
Action:

How I felt:
===

(   ) *Notes:*
Colour: **GREEN**
Word:
Meaning:
Action:

How I felt:
===

(   ) *Notes:*
Colour: **WHITE**
Word:
Meaning:
Action:

How I felt:
===

(   ) *Notes:*
Colour: **PINK**
Word:
Meaning:
Action:

How I felt:
===

(   ) *Notes:*
Colour: **BLUE**
Word:
Meaning:
Action:

How I felt:
===

(   ) *Notes:*
Colour: **BLACK**
Word:
Meaning:
Action:

How I felt:
===

(   ) *Notes:*
Colour: **RED**
Word:
Meaning:
Action:

How I felt:
===

Focus words for week 23 (Date   )

(   ) *Notes:*
Colour: `YELLOW`
Word:
Meaning:
Action:

How I felt:
==
(   ) *Notes:*
Colour: `GREEN`
Word:
Meaning:
Action:

How I felt:
==
(   ) *Notes:*
Colour: `WHITE`
Word:
Meaning:
Action:

How I felt:
==
(   ) *Notes:*
Colour: `PINK`
Word:
Meaning:
Action:

How I felt:
==
(   ) *Notes:*
Colour: `BLUE`
Word:
Meaning:
Action:

How I felt:
==
(   ) *Notes:*
Colour: `BLACK`
Word:
Meaning:
Action:

How I felt:
==
(   ) *Notes:*
Colour: `RED`
Word:
Meaning:
Action:

How I felt:
==

Focus words for week 24 (Date   )

( ) *Notes:*
Colour: **YELLOW**
Word:
Meaning:
Action:

How I felt:
===

( ) *Notes:*
Colour: **GREEN**
Word:
Meaning:
Action:

How I felt:
===

( ) *Notes:*
Colour: **WHITE**
Word:
Meaning:
Action:

How I felt:
===

( ) *Notes:*
Colour: **PINK**
Word:
Meaning:
Action:

How I felt:
===

( ) *Notes:*
Colour: **BLUE**
Word:
Meaning:
Action:

How I felt:
===

( ) *Notes:*
Colour: **BLACK**
Word:
Meaning:
Action:

How I felt:
===

( ) *Notes:*
Colour: **RED**
Word:
Meaning:
Action:

How I felt:
===

Summary/Intention (Date   )

Focus words for week 25 (Date   )

(   ) *Notes:*
Colour: **GREEN**
Word:
Meaning:
Action:

How I felt:

==

(   ) *Notes:*
Colour: **WHITE**
Word:
Meaning:
Action:

How I felt:

==

(   ) *Notes:*
Colour: **RED**
Word:
Meaning:
Action:

How I felt:

==

(   ) *Notes:*
Colour: **BLUE**
Word:
Meaning:
Action:

How I felt:

==

(   ) *Notes:*
Colour: **BLACK**
Word:
Meaning:
Action:

How I felt:

==

(   ) *Notes:*
Colour: **YELLOW**
Word:
Meaning:
Action:

How I felt:

==

(   ) *Notes:*
Colour: **PINK**
Word:
Meaning:
Action:

How I felt:

==

( ) *Notes:*
Colour: `GREEN`
Word:
Meaning:
Action:

How I felt:
===

( ) *Notes:*
Colour: `WHITE`
Word:
Meaning:
Action:

How I felt:
===

( ) *Notes:*
Colour: `RED`
Word:
Meaning:
Action:

How I felt:
===

( ) *Notes:*
Colour: `BLUE`
Word:
Meaning:
Action:

How I felt:
===

( ) *Notes:*
Colour: `BLACK`
Word:
Meaning:
Action:

How I felt:
===

( ) *Notes:*
Colour: `YELLOW`
Word:
Meaning:
Action:

How I felt:
===

( ) *Notes:*
Colour: `PINK`
Word:
Meaning:
Action:

How I felt:
===

Focus words for week 27 (Date   )

(   ) *Notes:*
Colour: **GREEN**
Word:
Meaning:
Action:

How I felt:
===

(   ) *Notes:*
Colour: **WHITE**
Word:
Meaning:
Action:

How I felt:
===

(   ) *Notes:*
Colour: **RED**
Word:
Meaning:
Action:

How I felt:
===

(   ) *Notes:*
Colour: **BLUE**
Word:
Meaning:
Action:

How I felt:
===

(   ) *Notes:*
Colour: **BLACK**
Word:
Meaning:
Action:

How I felt:
===

(   ) *Notes:*
Colour: **YELLOW**
Word:
Meaning:
Action:

How I felt:
===

(   ) *Notes:*
Colour: **PINK**
Word:
Meaning:
Action:

How I felt:
===

Focus words for week 28 (Date   )

(   ) *Notes:*
Colour: GREEN
Word:
Meaning:
Action:

How I felt:

==

(   ) *Notes:*
Colour: WHITE
Word:
Meaning:
Action:

How I felt:

==

(   ) *Notes:*
Colour: RED
Word:
Meaning:
Action:

How I felt:

==

(   ) *Notes:*
Colour: BLUE
Word:
Meaning:
Action:

How I felt:

==

(   ) *Notes:*
Colour: BLACK
Word:
Meaning:
Action:

How I felt:

==

(   ) *Notes:*
Colour: YELLOW
Word:
Meaning:
Action:

How I felt:

==

(   ) *Notes:*
Colour: PINK
Word:
Meaning:
Action:

How I felt:

==

Summary/Intention (Date   )

Focus words for week 29 (Date   )

(   ) *Notes:*
Colour: `GREEN`
Word:
Meaning:
Action:

How I felt:

===

(   ) *Notes:*
Colour: `BLUE`
Word:
Meaning:
Action:

How I felt:

===

(   ) *Notes:*
Colour: `PINK`
Word:
Meaning:
Action:

How I felt:

===

(   ) *Notes:*
Colour: `YELLOW`
Word:
Meaning:
Action:

How I felt:

===

(   ) *Notes:*
Colour: `RED`
Word:
Meaning:
Action:

How I felt:

===

(   ) *Notes:*
Colour: `WHITE`
Word:
Meaning:
Action:

How I felt:

===

(   ) *Notes:*
Colour: `BLACK`
Word:
Meaning:
Action:

How I felt:

===

Focus words for week 30 (Date   )

( ) *Notes:*
Colour: **GREEN**
Word:
Meaning:
Action:

How I felt:
===

( ) *Notes:*
Colour: **BLUE**
Word:
Meaning:
Action:

How I felt:
===

( ) *Notes:*
Colour: **PINK**
Word:
Meaning:
Action:

How I felt:
===

( ) *Notes:*
Colour: **YELLOW**
Word:
Meaning:
Action:

How I felt:
===

( ) *Notes:*
Colour: **RED**
Word:
Meaning:
Action:

How I felt:
===

( ) *Notes:*
Colour: **WHITE**
Word:
Meaning:
Action:

How I felt:
===

( ) *Notes:*
Colour: **BLACK**
Word:
Meaning:
Action:

How I felt:
===

Focus words for week 31 (Date   )

(   ) *Notes:*
Colour: **GREEN**
Word:
Meaning:
Action:

How I felt:
===

(   ) *Notes:*
Colour: **BLUE**
Word:
Meaning:
Action:

How I felt:
===

(   ) *Notes:*
Colour: **PINK**
Word:
Meaning:
Action:

How I felt:
===

(   ) *Notes:*
Colour: **YELLOW**
Word:
Meaning:
Action:

How I felt:
===

(   ) *Notes:*
Colour: **RED**
Word:
Meaning:
Action:

How I felt:
===

(   ) *Notes:*
Colour: **WHITE**
Word:
Meaning:
Action:

How I felt:
===

(   ) *Notes:*
Colour: **BLACK**
Word:
Meaning:
Action:

How I felt:
===

(   ) *Notes:*
Colour: **GREEN**
Word:
Meaning:
Action:

How I felt:
===

(   ) *Notes:*
Colour: **BLUE**
Word:
Meaning:
Action:

How I felt:
===

(   ) *Notes:*
Colour: **PINK**
Word:
Meaning:
Action:

How I felt:
===

(   ) *Notes:*
Colour: **YELLOW**
Word:
Meaning:
Action:

How I felt:
===

(   ) *Notes:*
Colour: **RED**
Word:
Meaning:
Action:

How I felt:
===

(   ) *Notes:*
Colour: **WHITE**
Word:
Meaning:
Action:

How I felt:
===

(   ) *Notes:*
Colour: **BLACK**
Word:
Meaning:
Action:

How I felt:
===

Summary/Intention (Date   )

Focus words for week 33 (Date   )

(   ) *Notes:*
Colour: **PINK**
Word:
Meaning:
Action:

How I felt:
===

(   ) *Notes:*
Colour: **RED**
Word:
Meaning:
Action:

How I felt:
===

(   ) *Notes:*
Colour: **WHITE**
Word:
Meaning:
Action:

How I felt:
===

(   ) *Notes:*
Colour: **BLACK**
Word:
Meaning:
Action:

How I felt:
===

(   ) *Notes:*
Colour: **BLUE**
Word:
Meaning:
Action:

How I felt:
===

(   ) *Notes:*
Colour: **YELLOW**
Word:
Meaning:
Action:

How I felt:
===

(   ) *Notes:*
Colour: **GREEN**
Word:
Meaning:
Action:

How I felt:
===

Focus words for week 34 (Date   )

(   ) *Notes:*
Colour: **PINK**
Word:
Meaning:
Action:

How I felt:

===

(   ) *Notes:*
Colour: **RED**
Word:
Meaning:
Action:

How I felt:

===

(   ) *Notes:*
Colour: **WHITE**
Word:
Meaning:
Action:

How I felt:

===

(   ) *Notes:*
Colour: **BLACK**
Word:
Meaning:
Action:

How I felt:

===

(   ) *Notes:*
Colour: **BLUE**
Word:
Meaning:
Action:

How I felt:

===

(   ) *Notes:*
Colour: **YELLOW**
Word:
Meaning:
Action:

How I felt:

===

(   ) *Notes:*
Colour: **GREEN**
Word:
Meaning:
Action:

How I felt:

===

(   ) *Notes:*
Colour: **PINK**
Word:
Meaning:
Action:

How I felt:
===

(   ) *Notes:*
Colour: **RED**
Word:
Meaning:
Action:

How I felt:
===

(   ) *Notes:*
Colour: **WHITE**
Word:
Meaning:
Action:

How I felt:
===

(   ) *Notes:*
Colour: **BLACK**
Word:
Meaning:
Action:

How I felt:
===

(   ) *Notes:*
Colour: **BLUE**
Word:
Meaning:
Action:

How I felt:
===

(   ) *Notes:*
Colour: **YELLOW**
Word:
Meaning:
Action:

How I felt:
===

(   ) *Notes:*
Colour: **GREEN**
Word:
Meaning:
Action:

How I felt:
===

(   ) *Notes:*
Colour: **PINK**
Word:
Meaning:
Action:

How I felt:

==

(   ) *Notes:*
Colour: **RED**
Word:
Meaning:
Action:

How I felt:

==

(   ) *Notes:*
Colour: **WHITE**
Word:
Meaning:
Action:

How I felt:

==

(   ) *Notes:*
Colour: **BLACK**
Word:
Meaning:
Action:

How I felt:

==

(   ) *Notes:*
Colour: **BLUE**
Word:
Meaning:
Action:

How I felt:

==

(   ) *Notes:*
Colour: **YELLOW**
Word:
Meaning:
Action:

How I felt:

==

(   ) *Notes:*
Colour: **GREEN**
Word:
Meaning:
Action:

How I felt:

==

Summary/Intention (Date   )

Focus words for week 37 (Date   )

(   ) *Notes:*
Colour: **RED**
Word:
Meaning:
Action:

How I felt:

===

(   ) *Notes:*
Colour: **BLUE**
Word:
Meaning:
Action:

How I felt:

===

(   ) *Notes:*
Colour: **BLACK**
Word:
Meaning:
Action:

How I felt:

===

(   ) *Notes:*
Colour: **YELLOW**
Word:
Meaning:
Action:

How I felt:

===

(   ) *Notes:*
Colour: **PINK**
Word:
Meaning:
Action:

How I felt:

===

(   ) *Notes:*
Colour: **GREEN**
Word:
Meaning:
Action:

How I felt:

===

(   ) *Notes:*
Colour: **WHITE**
Word:
Meaning:
Action:

How I felt:

===

(   ) *Notes:*
Colour: **RED**
Word:
Meaning:
Action:

How I felt:
===

(   ) *Notes:*
Colour: **BLUE**
Word:
Meaning:
Action:

How I felt:
===

(   ) *Notes:*
Colour: **BLACK**
Word:
Meaning:
Action:

How I felt:
===

(   ) *Notes:*
Colour: **YELLOW**
Word:
Meaning:
Action:

How I felt:
===

(   ) *Notes:*
Colour: **PINK**
Word:
Meaning:
Action:

How I felt:
===

(   ) *Notes:*
Colour: **GREEN**
Word:
Meaning:
Action:

How I felt:
===

(   ) *Notes:*
Colour: **WHITE**
Word:
Meaning:
Action:

How I felt:
===

Focus words for week 39 (Date   )

(   ) *Notes:*
Colour: `RED`
Word:
Meaning:
Action:

How I felt:
===

(   ) *Notes:*
Colour: `BLUE`
Word:
Meaning:
Action:

How I felt:
===

(   ) *Notes:*
Colour: `BLACK`
Word:
Meaning:
Action:

How I felt:
===

(   ) *Notes:*
Colour: `YELLOW`
Word:
Meaning:
Action:

How I felt:
===

(   ) *Notes:*
Colour: `PINK`
Word:
Meaning:
Action:

How I felt:
===

(   ) *Notes:*
Colour: `GREEN`
Word:
Meaning:
Action:

How I felt:
===

(   ) *Notes:*
Colour: `WHITE`
Word:
Meaning:
Action:

How I felt:
===

Focus words for week 40 (Date   )

(   ) *Notes:*
Colour: `RED`
Word:
Meaning:
Action:

How I felt:
==

(   ) *Notes:*
Colour: `BLUE`
Word:
Meaning:
Action:

How I felt:
==

(   ) *Notes:*
Colour: `BLACK`
Word:
Meaning:
Action:

How I felt:
==

(   ) *Notes:*
Colour: `YELLOW`
Word:
Meaning:
Action:

How I felt:
==

(   ) *Notes:*
Colour: `PINK`
Word:
Meaning:
Action:

How I felt:
==

(   ) *Notes:*
Colour: `GREEN`
Word:
Meaning:
Action:

How I felt:
==

(   ) *Notes:*
Colour: `WHITE`
Word:
Meaning:
Action:

How I felt:
==

Summary/Intention (Date   )

Focus words for week 41 (Date   )

(   ) *Notes:*
Colour: **YELLOW**
Word:
Meaning:
Action:

How I felt:
==

(   ) *Notes:*
Colour: **RED**
Word:
Meaning:
Action:

How I felt:
==

(   ) *Notes:*
Colour: **WHITE**
Word:
Meaning:
Action:

How I felt:
==

(   ) *Notes:*
Colour: **BLUE**
Word:
Meaning:
Action:

How I felt:
==

(   ) *Notes:*
Colour: **BLACK**
Word:
Meaning:
Action:

How I felt:
==

(   ) *Notes:*
Colour: **GREEN**
Word:
Meaning:
Action:

How I felt:
==

(   ) *Notes:*
Colour: **PINK**
Word:
Meaning:
Action:

How I felt:
==

Focus words for week 42 (Date   )

(   ) *Notes:*
Colour: **YELLOW**
Word:
Meaning:
Action:

How I felt:

==

(   ) *Notes:*
Colour: **RED**
Word:
Meaning:
Action:

How I felt:

==

(   ) *Notes:*
Colour: **WHITE**
Word:
Meaning:
Action:

How I felt:

==

(   ) *Notes:*
Colour: **BLUE**
Word:
Meaning:
Action:

How I felt:

==

(   ) *Notes:*
Colour: **BLACK**
Word:
Meaning:
Action:

How I felt:

==

(   ) *Notes:*
Colour: **GREEN**
Word:
Meaning:
Action:

How I felt:

==

(   ) *Notes:*
Colour: **PINK**
Word:
Meaning:
Action:

How I felt:

==

Focus words for week 43 (Date   )

(   ) *Notes:*
Colour: `YELLOW`
Word:
Meaning:
Action:

How I felt:
===

(   ) *Notes:*
Colour: `RED`
Word:
Meaning:
Action:

How I felt:
===

(   ) *Notes:*
Colour: `WHITE`
Word:
Meaning:
Action:

How I felt:
===

(   ) *Notes:*
Colour: `BLUE`
Word:
Meaning:
Action:

How I felt:
===

(   ) *Notes:*
Colour: `BLACK`
Word:
Meaning:
Action:

How I felt:
===

(   ) *Notes:*
Colour: `GREEN`
Word:
Meaning:
Action:

How I felt:
===

(   ) *Notes:*
Colour: `PINK`
Word:
Meaning:
Action:

How I felt:
===

(   ) *Notes:*
Colour: **YELLOW**
Word:
Meaning:
Action:

How I felt:
===

(   ) *Notes:*
Colour: **RED**
Word:
Meaning:
Action:

How I felt:
===

(   ) *Notes:*
Colour: **WHITE**
Word:
Meaning:
Action:

How I felt:
===

(   ) *Notes:*
Colour: **BLUE**
Word:
Meaning:
Action:

How I felt:
===

(   ) *Notes:*
Colour: **BLACK**
Word:
Meaning:
Action:

How I felt:
===

(   ) *Notes:*
Colour: **GREEN**
Word:
Meaning:
Action:

How I felt:
===

(   ) *Notes:*
Colour: **PINK**
Word:
Meaning:
Action:

How I felt:
===

Summary/Intention (Date   )

Focus words for week 45 (Date   )

(   ) *Notes:*
Colour: **BLUE**
Word:
Meaning:
Action:

How I felt:
==

(   ) *Notes:*
Colour: **GREEN**
Word:
Meaning:
Action:

How I felt:
==

(   ) *Notes:*
Colour: **PINK**
Word:
Meaning:
Action:

How I felt:
==

(   ) *Notes:*
Colour: **WHITE**
Word:
Meaning:
Action:

How I felt:
==

(   ) *Notes:*
Colour: **BLACK**
Word:
Meaning:
Action:

How I felt:
==

(   ) *Notes:*
Colour: **YELLOW**
Word:
Meaning:
Action:

How I felt:
==

(   ) *Notes:*
Colour: **RED**
Word:
Meaning:
Action:

How I felt:
==

Focus words for week 46 (Date   )

(   ) *Notes:*
Colour: BLUE
Word:
Meaning:
Action:

How I felt:
==

(   ) *Notes:*
Colour: GREEN
Word:
Meaning:
Action:

How I felt:
==

(   ) *Notes:*
Colour: PINK
Word:
Meaning:
Action:

How I felt:
==

(   ) *Notes:*
Colour: WHITE
Word:
Meaning:
Action:

How I felt:
==

(   ) *Notes:*
Colour: BLACK
Word:
Meaning:
Action:

How I felt:
==

(   ) *Notes:*
Colour: YELLOW
Word:
Meaning:
Action:

How I felt:
==

(   ) *Notes:*
Colour: RED
Word:
Meaning:
Action:

How I felt:
==

Focus words for week 47 (Date   )

(   ) *Notes:*
Colour: **BLUE**
Word:
Meaning:
Action:

How I felt:
==

(   ) *Notes:*
Colour: **GREEN**
Word:
Meaning:
Action:

How I felt:
==

(   ) *Notes:*
Colour: **PINK**
Word:
Meaning:
Action:

How I felt:
==

(   ) *Notes:*
Colour: **WHITE**
Word:
Meaning:
Action:

How I felt:
==

(   ) *Notes:*
Colour: **BLACK**
Word:
Meaning:
Action:

How I felt:
==

(   ) *Notes:*
Colour: **YELLOW**
Word:
Meaning:
Action:

How I felt:
==

(   ) *Notes:*
Colour: **RED**
Word:
Meaning:
Action:

How I felt:
==

Focus words for week 48 (Date   )

(   ) *Notes:*

Colour: **BLUE**

Word:

Meaning:

Action:

How I felt:

==

(   ) *Notes:*

Colour: **GREEN**

Word:

Meaning:

Action:

How I felt:

==

(   ) *Notes:*

Colour: **PINK**

Word:

Meaning:

Action:

How I felt:

==

(   ) *Notes:*

Colour: **WHITE**

Word:

Meaning:

Action:

How I felt:

==

(   ) *Notes:*

Colour: **BLACK**

Word:

Meaning:

Action:

How I felt:

==

(   ) *Notes:*

Colour: **YELLOW**

Word:

Meaning:

Action:

How I felt:

==

(   ) *Notes:*

Colour: **RED**

Word:

Meaning:

Action:

How I felt:

==

Summary/Intention (Date   )

Focus words for week 49 (Date   )

(   ) *Notes:*
Colour: `GREEN`
Word:
Meaning:
Action:

How I felt:
===

(   ) *Notes:*
Colour: `BLUE`
Word:
Meaning:
Action:

How I felt:
===

(   ) *Notes:*
Colour: `PINK`
Word:
Meaning:
Action:

How I felt:
===

(   ) *Notes:*
Colour: `YELLOW`
Word:
Meaning:
Action:

How I felt:
===

(   ) *Notes:*
Colour: `RED`
Word:
Meaning:
Action:

How I felt:
===

(   ) *Notes:*
Colour: `WHITE`
Word:
Meaning:
Action:

How I felt:
===

(   ) *Notes:*
Colour: `BLACK`
Word:
Meaning:
Action:

How I felt:
===

Focus words for week 50 (Date   )

(   ) *Notes:*
Colour: **RED**
Word:
Meaning:
Action:

How I felt:
==

(   ) *Notes:*
Colour: **GREEN**
Word:
Meaning:
Action:

How I felt:
==

(   ) *Notes:*
Colour: **BLUE**
Word:
Meaning:
Action:

How I felt:
==

(   ) *Notes:*
Colour: **WHITE**
Word:
Meaning:
Action:

How I felt:
==

(   ) *Notes:*
Colour: **BLACK**
Word:
Meaning:
Action:

How I felt:
==

(   ) *Notes:*
Colour: **PINK**
Word:
Meaning:
Action:

How I felt:
==

(   ) *Notes:*
Colour: **YELLOW**
Word:
Meaning:
Action:

How I felt:
==

(   ) *Notes:*
Colour: BLUE
Word:
Meaning:
Action:

How I felt:
===

(   ) *Notes:*
Colour: YELLOW
Word:
Meaning:
Action:

How I felt:
===

(   ) *Notes:*
Colour: GREEN
Word:
Meaning:
Action:

How I felt:
===

(   ) *Notes:*
Colour: PINK
Word:
Meaning:
Action:

How I felt:
===

(   ) *Notes:*
Colour: BLACK
Word:
Meaning:
Action:

How I felt:
===

(   ) *Notes:*
Colour: WHITE
Word:
Meaning:
Action:

How I felt:
===

(   ) *Notes:*
Colour: RED
Word:
Meaning:
Action:

How I felt:
===

(   ) *Notes:*
Colour: WHITE
Word:
Meaning:
Action:

How I felt:
==

(   ) *Notes:*
Colour: RED
Word:
Meaning:
Action:

How I felt:
==

(   ) *Notes:*
Colour: YELLOW
Word:
Meaning:
Action:

How I felt:
==

(   ) *Notes:*
Colour: GREEN
Word:
Meaning:
Action:

How I felt:
==

(   ) *Notes:*
Colour: BLUE
Word:
Meaning:
Action:

How I felt:
==

(   ) *Notes:*
Colour: BLACK
Word:
Meaning:
Action:

How I felt:
==

(   ) *Notes:*
Colour: PINK
Word:
Meaning:
Action:

How I felt:
==

Summary/Intention (Date   )

Final Summary

Phone Numbers and Important Information